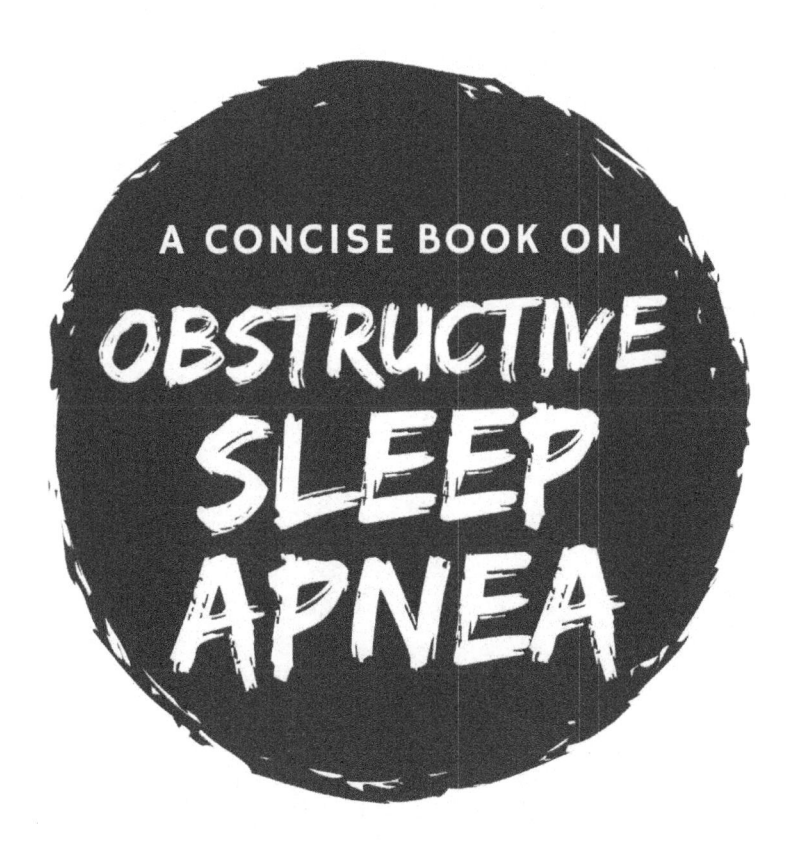

A CONCISE BOOK ON OBSTRUCTIVE SLEEP APNEA

A CONCISE BOOK ON

OBSTRUCTIVE SLEEP APNEA

Dr. Mrityunjay Sharma, MD
Dr. Deepanjali Sharma, MD

ISBN: 9798702142029

Copyright © 2021 Dr. Mrityunjay Sharma and Dr. Deepanjali Sharma. All rights reserved.
No part of this book may be reproduced, or stored in a retrieval system, or transmitted in any form or by any means, electronic, mechanical, photocopying, recording, or otherwise, without express written permission of the publisher.

Cover design by: Ayan Sharma
Model: Ayush Sharma
Picture Credit: Shahnawaz Ahmed

Contents

Preface 1
Chapter: 1 Sleep 3
    Introduction 3
    Sleep cycle and regulation 4
    Sleep stages 6
Chapter 2: Sleep-related breathing disorders 9
    ICSD classification 9
    Definitions 10
Chapter 3: Obstructive Sleep Apnea 12
    Introduction 12
    Epidemiology of OSA 12
    Risk Factors 13
    Etiology and Pathophysiology 14
Chapter 4: Association of OSA with Obesity and Type 2 Diabetes Mellitus 18
    Obesity 18
    Type 2 Diabetes Mellitus 21
    Association between OSA and T2DM 23
Chapter 5: Clinical Features (Signs and symptoms) 27
    Physical Examination 28
Chapter 6: Screening 29
    STOP-BANG (8-item questionnaire): 29
    Epworth sleepiness scale: 31

Chapter 7: Diagnosis 34
Chapter 8: Polysomnography 39
Chapter 9: Consequences of OSA 45
Chapter 10: Management 49
    General measures 49
    Weight loss 49
    Noninvasive ventilation 50
    CPAP (Continuous Positive Airway Pressure) therapy 52
    BPAP therapy (Bi-level Positive Airway Pressure) 58
    Oral appliances 58
    Surgical Approaches 61
    Medications 66
Chapter: 11 Prevention 69
    Prevention 69
Chapter 12: Follow up 70
Chapter 13: Role of yoga 71
Chapter 14: Role of reflexology acupressure and acupuncture 79

Preface

Obstructive Sleep Apnea is an important yet potentially serious medical condition that has become increasingly common for the past 50 years. The ever-increasing high prevalence of Obstructive sleep apnea and its substantial role in significant morbidities have greatly intensified the need to identify and correctly manage obstructive sleep apnea syndrome.

It is our hope that this book will provide a practical, updated and rapid reference for undergraduates, interns, postgraduates and health professionals who deal with obstructive sleep apnea as a text or as patients on a regular basis in outpatient as well as inpatient settings. This book aims to serve as a first-line reference in a very portable form that can be carried around and used as a quick and easy guide all the while presenting its readers with a clear and concise message on how to best identify, investigate and manage the condition with the best recommended clinical as well as non-clinical approaches.

Dr. Mrityunjay Sharma
Dr. Deepanjali Sharma

This page is intentionally left blank.

Chapter: 1 Sleep

Introduction

"Each night, when I go to sleep, I die. And the next morning, when I wake up, I am reborn." — Mahatma Gandhi.

"Your future depends on your dreams, so go to sleep." – Mesut Barazany.

Essentially every individual sleeps and leaves cognizance behind and lives a dream for quite a long time every night and every morning when he/she wakes up, he/she might or might not recollect things recently passed. In simple words, sleep reboots your brain and mind. All organisms exhibit a characteristic sleep-wake pattern.

"Sleep is a reversible physiological state which exhibits a period of reduced responsiveness to stimuli and is characterized by typical discharge of neuronal signals and neurotransmitters."

Sleep plays a vital role in shaping your perfect health. Sleep deficiency may increase cardiovascular, metabolic, and cerebrovascular events.

Regulatory centers in the brain and neurotransmitters (neuro-signaling chemicals) control sleep by switching off and on brain activities.

Sleep cycle and regulation

Sleep is a complex but essential and irreplaceable aspect of human biology. There is much to be determined about the structures, processes, and pathways of sleep regulation and sleep relationship to daytime functioning and overall well-being.

Sleep and circadian rhythm are exceptionally coupled cycles and was depicted by Borbely et al. They defined the connection between circadian cycle (Process C) with the sleep cycle (Process S). The conducting state of an individual is governed by the connection between these two cycles (Figure 1.1).

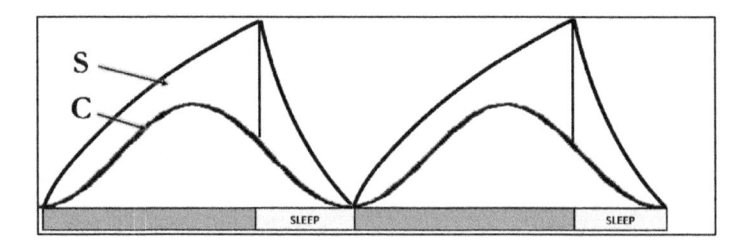

Figure 1.1: C- Biological clock; S- Sleep cycle

The drive for sleep, at a very low level just after sleep, increases progressively as wakefulness proceeds. In the evening, the alertness signal declines, and sleep drive becomes unopposed, and the sleep ensues.

A broad organization of subcortical structures and pathways is important to look after wakefulness.

Excitatory neurotransmitters like norepinephrine, serotonin, dopamine, histamine, acetylcholine, and orexin keep an individual active and awake. Deficiency or selective loss of such transmitters may cause Narcolepsy (excessive daytime sleepiness, fragmented sleep, and cataplexy). One of the commonest examples is the deficiency of orexin neurotransmitters in the forebrain due to the selective loss of orexin releasing neurons.

The ventrolateral preoptic area (VLPO) consists of inhibitory neurotransmitter releasing neurons, which suppress the activity of the arousal system (Figure 1.2). This mechanism induces and maintains sleep throughout. A faulty mechanism causes sleep-related disorders.

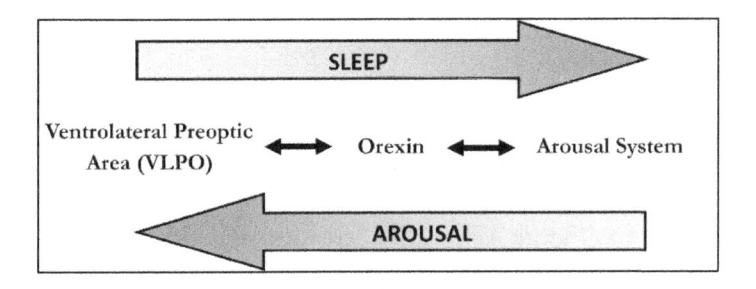

Figure 1.2: Ventrolateral preoptic area is releasing inhibitory neurotransmitter, which are suppressing the activity of the arousal system and inducing sleep.

Sleep and its stages are divided into two major types—non-rapid eye movement (NREM) sleep and rapid eye movement (REM) sleep. They switch with each other during sleep.

There are monoaminergic neurons and cholinergic neurons in the brainstem that inhibit each other reciprocally, and due to this phenomenon switching between NREM and REM sleep occurs.

REM-on cholinergic neurons are most active during REM sleep and while monoaminergic neurons remain less active or virtually silent, and this is how the switching between NREM and REM cycles during sleep takes place.

Sleep stages

REM sleep is characterized by:

- Active paralysis of muscles except for the diaphragm
- Autonomic instability leading to variation in heart rate and respiration
- Dreaming

Active paralysis of muscles prevents living out the dreams.

NREM sleep (Figure 1.4) is divided into stages N1, N2, and N3 based on the electroencephalogram. Earlier it was divided into N1, N2, N3, and N4 stages. In the stage 2 recording, a characteristic K complex and the sleep spindles are found.

During sleep, cycles have approximately a 90-minute duration, with REM sleep episodes occurring every 90 minutes. Episodes of REM sleep get longer and more phasic as the night progresses.

The **waking state** with the eyes open- High-frequency (15–60 Hz) and low-amplitude activity (~30 μV) activity, also known as a beta activity.

Stage I- Decreasing EEG frequency (4–8 Hz) and increasing amplitude (50–100 μV), also known as theta waves.

Stage II- 10–15 Hz oscillations (50–150 μV), also known as spindles. K complex is seen in this stage of sleep. (Figure 1. 3)

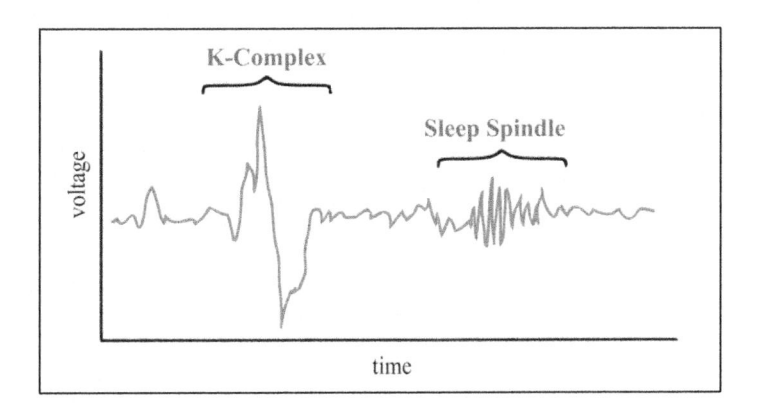

Figure 1.3: Showing K- complex and sleep spindle

Stage III- Slower waves at 2–4 Hz (100–150 μV).

Stage IV- Slow waves at 0.5–2 Hz (100–200 μV), also known as delta waves.

REM sleep- Low-voltage, high-frequency activity similar to the EEG activity of individuals who are awake.

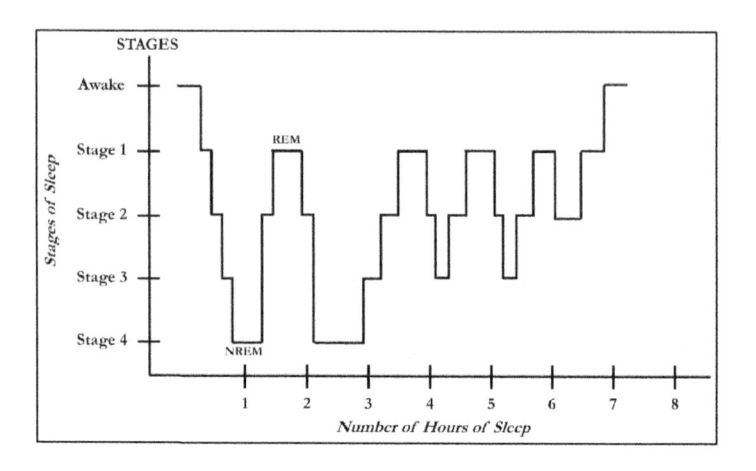

Figure 1.4: Stages of NREM

As you can see in the figure 1.4, the episodes of REM sleep become longer and regular as the night progresses.

Chapter 2: Sleep-related breathing disorders

It is a common medical disorder characterized by abnormal respiration during sleep. SDB was first reported in the 19th century, but in the last 40 years, pathogenesis, diagnostic, and treatment modalities of sleep apnea have been well understood[9]. Terms obstructive sleep apnea syndrome (OSAS) and sleep apnea syndrome were coined by Guilleminault et al. in 1976.

ICSD classification

International Classification of Sleep Disorders is the most widely used classification system for sleep disorders. It includes seven major categories of sleep disorders.

1- Insomnia
    a. Chronic insomnia disorder
    b. Short- term insomnia disorder
2- Sleep-related breathing disorders
    a. Central sleep apnea syndrome
    b. Obstructive sleep apnea syndrome.
    c. Sleep-related hypoventilation syndrome
3- Central disorders of hypersomnolence
    a. Narcolepsy
    b. Idiopathic hypersomnia
    c. Klein- Levin syndrome

  d. Other hypersomnias
4- Circadian rhythm sleep-wake disorders
5- Parasomnias
  a. NREM related parasomnias
  b. REM related parasomnias
  c. Other parasomnias
6- Sleep-related movement disorders
  a. Restless leg syndrome
  b. Periodic limb movement disorders
7- Other sleep disorders

Definitions

Apneas- Episodes of breathing cessation for 10 seconds.

Hypopneas- Episodes of decrement in airflow.

RERA (Respiratory Effort–Related Arousal) -

Arousal from sleep without meeting the criteria of hypopnea or apnea characterized by breaths with increasing effort is known as RERA.

Apnea–hypopnea index (AHI) - Number of apneas and hypopneas per hour of sleep. It is used to describe the severity of sleep apnea.

Respiratory disturbance index (RDI) - Number of apneas, hypopneas, and RERAs per hour of sleep.

Obstructive Sleep Apnea – it is characterized by a repetitive, partial, or complete collapse of the upper airway during sleep. AHI ≥ 5 events/hour is the cut-off value for OSA, which includes obstructive or mixed events of more than 50% of the total events.

OSAS (Obstructive Sleep Apnea Syndrome) - an AHI ≥ 5 events/h with persistent symptoms like excessive daytime sleepiness, unrefreshing sleep, or tiredness.

Central Sleep Apnea- It is defined as repeated episodes of apnea in the absence of respiratory muscle effort.

Obesity Hypoventilation Syndrome (Pickwickian syndrome)- This is diagnosed once all other diseases have been excluded. The characteristic features are sleep-disordered breathing, obesity, hypoventilation, and daytime hypercapnia.

Chapter 3: Obstructive Sleep Apnea

Introduction

It is characterized by a repetitive, partial, or complete collapse of the upper airway during sleep. AHI ≥ 5 events/hour is the cut-off value for OSA, which includes obstructive or mixed events of more than 50% of the total events.

Classification- (Based on AHI)

Mild	5 to 15 AHI
Moderate	15 to 30 AHI
Severe	>30 events/h AHI

Epidemiology of OSA

The prevalence of OSA is dependent on several factors. It depends upon the Type of parameters used for the study. E.g., methods used for the measurement of sleep-disordered breathing, population characteristics (e.g., obesity, ethnicity), definitions used to define disease, and the threshold of AHI used to define OSA.

In the US, a community-based cohort study known as Wisconsin Sleep Cohort Study reports a 4% and 2% prevalence of OSA in males and females, respectively, between 30 and 60 years of age.

In India, the estimated prevalence of symptomatic OSA was to be between 3% and 8% in men and 1% and 5% in women. The prevalence of OSA in the Indian population is three-fold higher in men as compared to women. In the North Indian population, a study by Singh et al. found that 6.2% of the total population were at high risk of OSAS, whereas 33.5% of the obese population was at high-risk OSAS.

Studies suggest that the prevalence of OSA is two to three times higher in men than women. The risk for OSA increases threefold higher, approximately, in postmenopausal women compared to premenopausal women.

Differences in body fat distribution in males may be one of the reasons for the increased prevalence of OSA as males have relatively more central fat distribution, including the neck.

Studies show that the increased prevalence of OSA in the population through midlife achieves a plateau after 60 to 65 years of age.

The prevalence of OSA among Asians is similar to Caucasian population samples.

Risk Factors

Gender (male/female- 3:1)

Genetic factors/family history

Obesity (Body Mass Index > 30 kg/m2)

Neck size (Collar size >17 inches in males, >16 inches in females)

Upper airway and craniofacial anatomy

    Macroglossia

    Lateral peritonsillar narrowing

    Elongation/enlargement of the soft palate

    Tonsillar hypertrophy

    Nasal septal deviation

    Retrognathia, micrognathia

    Narrowing of the hard palate

Genetic disorders like Down syndrome

Endocrine disorders like Hypothyroidism, PCOS (polycystic ovarian syndrome), and Acromegaly

Etiology and Pathophysiology

It involves both anatomic and neurologic components.

Anatomic component-

The upper airway extending from the posterior margin of the nasal septum to the larynx lacks the bony rigid support and is divided into four following anatomic regions (Fig. 3.1 & 3.2).

• Nasopharynx: A potential space between the nares and the hard palate.

- Oropharynx (Retropalatal): A potential space between the hard palate and the posterior edge of the soft palate.

- Oropharynx (Retroglossal): A potential space between the posterior edge of the soft palate and the base of the epiglottis.

- Hypopharynx: A potential space from the base of the tongue to the larynx.

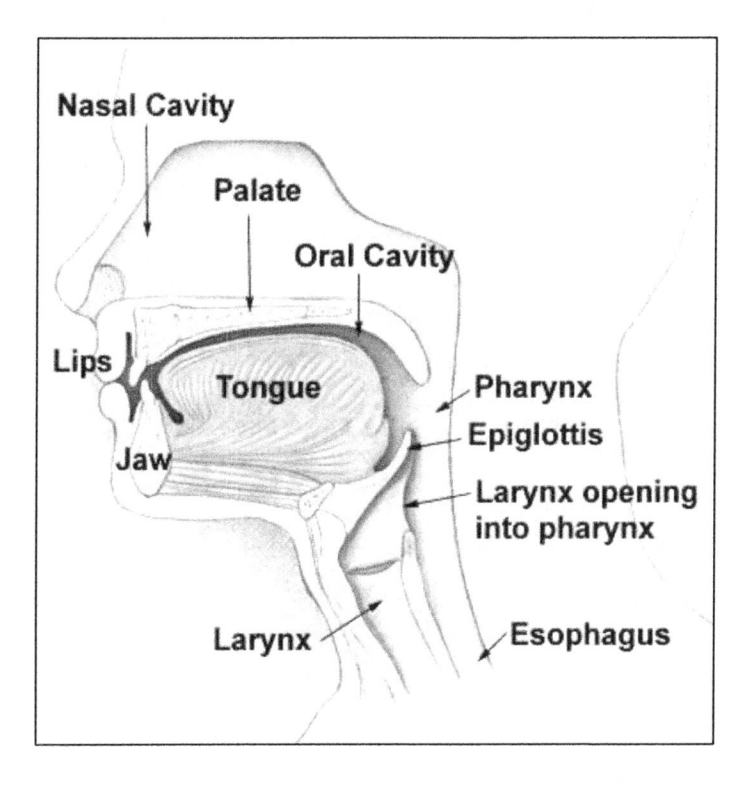

Fig. 3.1- Normal Anatomy

The extrathoracic upper airway remains at risk for collapse due to the lack of rigid support of cartilaginous rings, extraluminal pressure due to circumferential soft tissue structures, and negative pressure during inspiration. This pressure is offset by pharyngeal dilator muscles.

The size of the upper airway is very much affected by the transmural pressure. Numerically, transmural pressure is the difference between the pressure in the airway lumen and the pressure applied by the tissues surrounding it. Retropalatal and retroglossal regions are the most vulnerable regions for airway collapse.

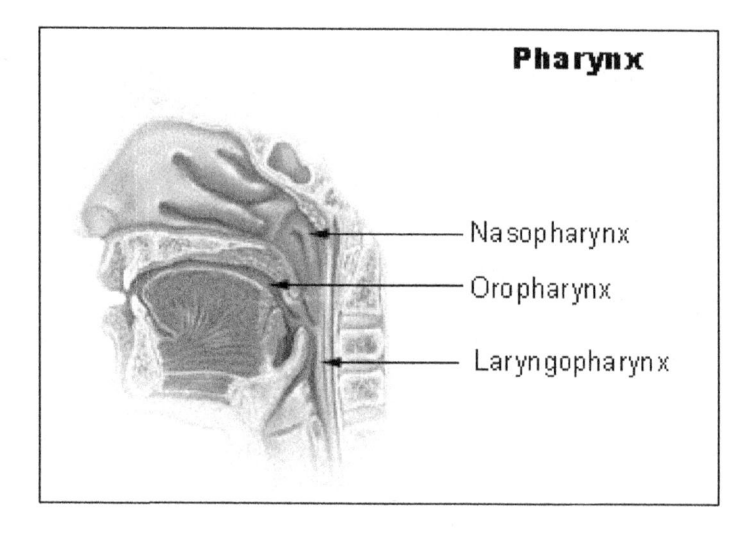

Figure 3.2: Showing subdivisions of pharynx

Among individuals, snoring, hypopneas and apneas are caused due to the collapse, which reduces the intraluminal diameter and increases the airway resistance.

Males are more susceptible to develop sleep apnea than females as males have larger pharyngeal airway cross-sectional area, longer airway length, and airway volumes, which make the airway more collapsible.

Neck circumference is found to be a strong predictor of OSA in population studies. It is found that patients with sleep apnea have longer soft palates, larger tongues, and excess upper airway soft tissue than normal subjects.

Neural component-

The nerve supply innervating the upper airway muscles involves many neurotransmitters, for example, norepinephrine, serotonin, GABA, orexin–acetylcholine that are influenced by sleep itself[24, 25] and it is seen that upper airway dilator muscle activity is reduced during sleep.

Genioglossus muscle activity reflex, which includes the activation of genioglossus via increased hypoglossal nerve discharge on detection of negative airway pressure by laryngeal mechanoreceptors, is diminished during NREM sleep, which is further reduced during the REM sleep, placing the airway at more risk for collapse. Recently, a novel, state sensitive motor inhibitory cholinergic channel has also been identified that operates at the hypoglossal motor pool as the principal mechanism of REM sleep pharyngeal motor inhibition[28].

Chapter 4: Association of OSA with Obesity and Type 2 Diabetes Mellitus

Obesity and Type 2 Diabetes Mellitus are one of the commonest prevalent diseases in society. Obstructive sleep apnea has been found commonly associated with these diseases. Due to a high prevalence and a common association of these diseases with OSA, they need a special mention here in this book.

Obesity

A state in which a person has accumulated excess adipose tissue mass.

Quantification of obesity-

- Body mass index (BMI)= weight/height^2 (in kg/m^2)
- Anthropometry- skinfold thickness
- Densitometry- underwater weighing

Intraabdominal and abdominal subcutaneous fat have more significance than subcutaneous fat present in the buttocks and lower extremities. For its determination, the waist-to-hip ratio is calculated. A ratio >0.9 in women and >1.0 in men is considered abnormal.

Obesity may be linked with several pulmonary abnormalities. It includes increased work of breathing, reduced chest wall compliance, increased minute ventilation, and reduced functional residual capacity and expiratory reserve volume, and obesity hypoventilation syndrome.

Pathogenesis of obesity and OSA

- Increased neck fat in obesity causes upper airway obstruction during sleep.
- Increased abdominal girth in a recumbent fashion decreases the lung volume in patients with obesity, which further worsens hypoxia during sleep.
- Neuronal dysfunction of the muscles in OSA may cause upper airway obstruction.
- Leptin hormone, produced by adipocyte tissue, plays a major role in appetite and metabolism regulation. Patients with leptin deficiency have more collapsible airways independent of weight. Obese patients are generally Leptin resistant and have high circulating levels of Leptin, rather than leptin deficiency.

BMIs for the midpoint of all heights and frames among both men and women range from 19 to 26 kg/m^2.

Ethnic-Specific Cutoff Values for Waist Circumference in South Asian population:

- Men > 90cm (>33.5 inches)
- Women > 80cm (>31.5 inches)

Craniofacial Anatomy-

Craniofacial features also play a role in non-obese individuals. Micrognathia, retroposed mandible, and narrowing of the hard palate are the primary risk factors for apnea in such patients.

Heritability of craniofacial abnormalities and upper airway soft tissue structures have also been observed in first-degree relatives and siblings. Examples are inferior displaced hyoid bone, retroposed mandible, lateral pharyngeal walls, tongue volume, and total soft tissue.

Endocrine Abnormalities

Thyroid disorders like the presence of a goiter may place the patient at risk for OSA. Thyroid surgeries like lobectomy or total thyroidectomy improve OSA symptoms like snoring and excessive somnolence in such patients. Hypothyroidism, when accompanied by Myxedema, is associated with both obstructive and central sleep apnea due to alterations in muscle function and blunted ventilatory response. Similarly, macroglossia associated with hypothyroidism also contributes to the development of OSA. In patients with

Acromegaly, OSA is common and often severe, presumably related to both osseous and soft tissue changes narrowing the upper airway.

Alcohol, sedatives, and hypnotics are detrimental for OSA as alcohol reduces the upper airway tone while sedatives or hypnotics affect the arousal mechanism.

Type 2 Diabetes Mellitus

Diabetes mellitus is a metabolic disorder that has the common phenotype of increased blood glucose level (hyperglycemia).

Interaction of genetics and environmental factors in Diabetes Mellitus causes metabolic dysregulation, which is associated with secondary pathophysiologic changes in multiple organ systems.

Classification:

On the basis of different pathogenic processes causing abnormal glucose homeostasis, diabetes mellitus is categorized into different forms. Broadly, there are two categories of diabetes mellitus and are designated as type 1 and type 2.

Type 1 DM- Complete or near-total insulin deficiency due to beta cell destruction. It may be immune-mediated or idiopathic.

Type 2 DM- Characterized by impaired insulin secretion, variable degrees of insulin resistance, and increased production of glucose.

Epidemiology

The worldwide prevalence of DM is rising gradually. In 1985 estimated cases of diabetes mellitus were 30 million, which reached 382 million in 2013, gradually.

As per International Diabetes Federation, the prevalence may rise up to 592 million by the year 2035. A sedentary lifestyle and increasing obesity are causing a more rapid increase in the prevalence of Type 2 DM worldwide. In India, the prevalence of Type 2 DM in 2013 was 65.1 million.

In individuals age >20 years prevalence of Type 2 DM is similar in men and women throughout most age ranges (14% and 11%, respectively).

Due to environmental, behavioral, and genetic factors prevalence of Type 2 DM varies in different geographical areas and in different ethnic populations within a country. Indigenous populations usually have a greater incidence of diabetes than the general population.

Criteria for the Diagnosis of Diabetes Mellitus

Any one of the followings:

• Symptoms of diabetes plus random blood glucose concentration ≥11.1 mmol/L (200 mg/dL)

• Fasting plasma glucose ≥7.0 mmol/L (126 mg/dL)

• Hemoglobin A1c (HbA1c) ≥ 6.5%

- 2-h plasma glucose ≥11.1 mmol/L (200 mg/dL) during an oral glucose tolerance test.

Management of Type 2 Diabetes Mellitus

The management primarily focuses on glycemic control, treatment of associated conditions, and prevention of complications. Glycemic control is done by improving diet, daily lifestyle modifications, and using oral or injectable medications. Screening of associated conditions like dyslipidemia, hypertension, obesity, coronary heart disease, or various complications of diabetes like retinopathy, cardiovascular disease, nephropathy, and neuropathy are looked for and managed accordingly.

Association between OSA and T2DM

Pathophysiology

Studies describe a two-way relationship between obstructive sleep apnea and Type 2 diabetes mellitus. A two-way relationship means that Type 2 diabetes mellitus is a risk factor for obstructive sleep apnea and obstructive sleep apnea is a risk factor for Type 2 diabetes mellitus.

It is found that there is a twofold increased rate of OSA in people with pre-diabetes and morbid obesity, compared to normoglycemic and morbidly obese patients.

Hypoxic episodes and sleep fragmentation in OSA cause several hormonal changes, which lead to activation of the sympathetic nervous system and the release of increased catecholamine, which causes glycogenesis and decreased insulin sensitivity. In addition, stimulation of the hypothalamic-pituitary-adrenal axis (HPA axis) releases increased levels of cortisol, which further impairs glucose metabolism by decreasing insulin release. Inflammatory processes due to oxidative stress and inflammatory markers (i.e., TNFα, IL-6) are also responsible for the development of the metabolic syndrome.

A low levels soluble leptin receptor has been reported in OSA, and due to which an increased level of free Leptin is also seen.

In a meta-analysis including 5953 patients with OSA, there were 332 incident cases who developed T2DM over 2-16 years duration. And the risk was greater in individuals with moderate to severe OSA.

Overweight or obese people with sleep-disordered breathing have a greater chance of developing diabetes when compared to overweight or people without sleep-disordered breathing.

Obese people with Type 2 Diabetes Mellitus who sleep for < 6.5 hours per night have a greater tendency to accumulate visceral fat and have increased levels of IL-6, IFN-γ, and TNF-α.

Patients with Type 2 Diabetes Mellitus are at increased risk of OSA, but many are undiagnosed. International Diabetes Federation Task

Force, 2008 issued a report on Epidemiology and Prevention that patients with T2DM should be assessed for OSA symptoms like snoring, daytime sleepiness, and apnoeic events.

There is evidence that glycemic control is associated with abnormalities of sleep in select populations. This is the other benefit of screening for OSA in people with diabetes.

It is observed in overnight polysomnography that in obese patients with Type 2 Diabetes Mellitus, the lowest oxygen saturation levels during sleep had the maximum percentage of the time, and also the severity of AHI was associated with increased postprandial glucose levels along with lower insulin sensitivity.

Association between untreated OSA and Glycemic Control in Type 2 Diabetic Patients

In a study by Aronsohn et al., 2010, full laboratory polysomnography (with a minimum laboratory recording time of 7h) was done on 60 patients with physician-diagnosed diabetes to assess the presence and severity of OSA. OSA severity was associated with poor glycemic control. Adjusted mean HbA1c was 7.3%, 7.7%, and 7.7% in mild, moderate, and severe OSA, respectively.

So as per evidence presence and severity of untreated OSA in type 2 diabetic patients may be associated with poorer glycemic control.

Based on these findings, reducing the severity of obstructive sleep apnea in patients may be an adjunctive therapeutic strategy for the optimization of glycemic control.

Chapter 5: Clinical Features (Signs and Symptoms)

Repetitive airway obstruction of the upper airway causes difficulty in breathing. Following are the symptoms patients of OSA usually present with.

- Loud snoring
- Unrefreshing sleep
- Excessive daytime sleepiness
- Choking or gasping episodes during sleep
- Observed apneas during sleep by partner
- Accidents while driving or during work
- Nocturnal awakening
- Nocturia
- Nocturnal sweating
- Irritability
- Lack of concentration
- Sometimes loss of libido or impotence.

Repetitive airway obstruction causes frequent nocturnal awakenings and sleep fragmentation, which leads to unrefreshed awakening and excessive daytime sleepiness. Unrefreshing sleep or unrefreshed awakening in the morning in untreated OSA is also attributed to decreased slow-wave sleep (non-REM stage 3), REM sleep, and more sleep stage transitions. People with OSA complain of sleepiness or drowsiness following meals, while watching television, reading, driving, or during a conversation. Lack of concentration and deficits in memory in individuals with untreated OSA affect the ability to function at work, which may cause depression and personality change.

Nocturia is attributed to increased Atrial Natriuretic Peptide (ANP) release in response to apnea-related right atrial stretch.

Physical Examination

A careful examination is needed in patients with suspected OSAS. The airway should be examined for its patency and anatomical abnormalities, for example, nasal obstruction due to asymmetry, polyps, mass, deviated nasal septum or hypertrophy of turbinates, craniofacial anomalies like micrognathia, mandibular retrognathia, etc., soft tissue abnormalities like macroglossia, tonsillar hypertrophy, lateral peritonsillar wall narrowing or enlarged uvula.

Measurement of height, weight, BMI, neck circumference, waist circumference is assessed for obesity. Measurements of blood pressure, blood sugar, and other systemic examination are also done for other associated comorbidities.

Neck circumference > 17 inches (43.2 cm) in males or > 16 inches (40.6 cm) in females have an increased risk for obstructive sleep apnea.

Chapter 6: Screening

Screening for Sleep Apnea

There have been many standardized instruments used for the risk stratification of sleep apnea.

1. Epworth Sleepiness Scale
2. Multivariable Apnea Prediction (MAP) Index
3. Berlin questionnaire
4. STOPBANG (8-item questionnaire)

The sensitivity and specificity of the Multivariable Apnea Prediction (MAP) Index and Berlin questionnaire questionnaires are variable in different populations.

STOP-BANG (8-item questionnaire):

STOP-BANG (8-item questionnaire) has a good predictive value for identifying severe OSA in the preoperative surgical setting. It is a quick, reliable, and easy-to-use screening tool.

It includes the following eight dichotomous parameters.

1. Snoring- yes/no
2. Tiredness- yes/no
3. Observed apneas- yes/no
4. Blood pressure- yes/no
5. Body Mass Index more than 35 kg/m2- yes/no
6. Age older than 50- yes/no

7. Neck circumference 16 inches / 40cm or large- yes/no
8. Gender (Male)- yes/no

The maximum score of this questionnaire is 8. The minimum score of this questionnaire is 0.

On the basis of scores obtained, patients can be classified into the following groups-

Risk of OSA according to STOP-Bang scores.

Low Risk:	0 - 2 points
Intermediate Risk:	3 - 4 points
High Risk:	5 - 8 points

Or

| Two or more points of 4 STOP questions + male gender |

Or

| 2 or more points of 4 STOP questions + BMI > 35kg/m2 |

The severity of OSA increases with an increase in stop bang score. The negative predictive value of this questionnaire is very high.

Limitations of STOP-BANG:

Selection bias

Manual error in measurements- for neck circumference

Epworth sleepiness scale:

This questionnaire is named after Epworth Hospital, situated in Melbourne.

It was first developed by Dr. Johns in 1990 for adults. This has been subsequently modified in further years.

This was developed with the intention to assess daytime sleepiness in patients by Dr. Johns.

Characteristics:

Small and easy to use

Eight questions

Self-administered questionnaire

Scores are given from 0 to 3 according to the chances of dozing off.

The score ranges from 0 to 24

The higher the ESS score, the higher will be the chances of daytime sleepiness.

Chances of dozing off or fallen asleep on a scale of 0 to 3 during different activities

The questionnaire includes:

1. Sitting and reading
2. Watching TV
3. Sitting inactive in a public place, such as a meeting or theatre
4. Riding as a passenger in a car for an hour without a break
5. Lying down to rest in the afternoon when circumstances permit
6. Sitting and talking to someone
7. Sitting quietly after a lunch without alcohol
8. Sitting in a car, stopped for a few minutes in traffic

ESS scores are interpreted as follows:

0-5- Lower Normal Daytime Sleepiness

6-10- Higher Normal Daytime Sleepiness

11-12- Excessive Daytime Sleepiness (Mild)

13-15- Excessive Daytime Sleepiness (Moderate)

16-24- Excessive Daytime Sleepiness (Severe)

Crash-risk while driving a car is high in people with ESS scores >15.

Limitations of ESS:

Subjective reports

Chances of biasing are more.

It cannot be used in isolation in legal implications.

Not a diagnostic tool

Not suitable for people with serious cognitive impairment

Cannot assess the circadian rhythm of sleep

Chapter 7: Diagnosis

Diagnosis of Obstructive Sleep Apnea

Gold standard diagnostic test for OSA is in-laboratory polysomnography (PSG), also known as Type I study. This test involves simultaneous recordings of multiple physiologic signals. On the basis of the number of signals, polysomnography is divided into four types or levels.

Level I includes EEG (electroencephalogram), EOG (electrooculogram), EMG (electromyogram), ECG (electrocardiogram), airflow, respiratory effort, O_2 saturation, videography in the presence of a lab attendant.

Level II includes seven channels- EEG, EOG, chin EMG, ECG/HR, airflow, O2 saturation, respiratory effort.

Level III includes four channels- ECG/HR, O2 saturation, airflow, and respiratory movement.

Level IV includes one or two channels- Airflow and/or O2 saturation.

EEG leads and other recordings are used to differentiate wakefulness from sleepiness and determines the different sleep stages. Respiratory effort is assessed by impedance plethysmography. Airflow changes are recorded by a probe, also known as a thermistor, which senses the temperature changes.

AHI (Apnea- hypopnea index)

The number of apneas and hypopneas per hour of sleep is used for the severity of sleep apnea.

AHI shows a linear relationship between the likelihood of adverse outcomes like strokes, hypertension, and itself, which makes it a useful determinant of OSA diagnosis.

Drawbacks:

It does not correlate with sleep quality measures and clinical outcomes[71].

It does not collect information regarding the nocturnal hypoxemia, degree of desaturation, hypoventilation (i.e., hypercapnia), or associated sleep disruption.

AHI (apnea-hypopnea index) and RDI (respiratory disturbance index) are commonly used for making a diagnosis of sleep-disordered breathing.

Apnea-Hypopnea Index (AHI)-

Calculated by the following formula:

Total number of episodes of apnea and hypopnea / Total numbers of hours of sleep

It can be defined as the "average number of episodes of apnea and hypopnea per hour."

Respiratory Disturbance Index-

Calculated by the following formula:

Total number of episodes of respiratory disturbances including apneas, hypopneas, and respiratory event-related arousals / Total numbers of hours of sleep

RDI can also be defined as the "average number of respiratory disturbances per hour."

American Academy of Sleep Medicine (AASM) is a leading professional society exclusively dedicated to sleep medicine. It sets standards and promotes research, education, and excellence in the field of sleep medicine.

Diagnostic criteria for OSA

For the diagnosis of OSA, at least 1 of the following criteria must be present:

1. More than five respiratory disturbances, including apneas, hypopneas, and respiratory effort-related arousals per hour of sleep and/or evidence of increased respiratory effort during each or all respiratory event.

The patient presenting with symptoms like excessive daytime somnolence, unrefreshing sleep, tiredness, loud snoring, insomnia, nighttime choking or gasping leading to arousals and/or unintentional naps during wakefulness

2. More than 15 respiratory disturbances, including apneas, hypopneas, respiratory effort-related arousals per hour of sleep, and/or evidence of respiratory effort during all or a portion of each respiratory event.

+/-

Patient presenting with symptoms like excessive daytime somnolence, unrefreshing sleep, tiredness, loud snoring, insomnia, nighttime choking or gasping leading to arousals and/or unintentional naps during wakefulness.

Other medical or neurologic disorders, use of medication, or substance abuse are excluded before making a diagnosis of OSA.

Differential diagnosis of OSA

Alveolar hypoventilation

Central sleep apnea

Cheyne-Stokes respiration

Idiopathic hypersomnia

Insufficient sleep

Laryngospasm due to gastroesophageal reflux

Narcolepsy

Obesity-hypoventilation syndrome (OHS or Pickwickian syndrome)

Panic attacks

Periodic limb movement disorder

Pulmonary edema related dyspnea

Simple snoring

Use of drug or substance abuse causing hypersomnia

Chapter 8: Polysomnography

Polysomnography is important for making a diagnosis of OSA and for the treatment benefit monitoring.

In- lab polysomnography with attended monitoring provides an additional benefit to diagnose periodic limb movements, a sleep-related behavioral disorder, etc.

Components of polysomnography

EEG (Electroencephalogram)

EOG (Electrooculogram)

Chin EMG (Electromyogram)

Anterior tibialis EMG (Electromyogram)

ECG (Electrocardiogram)

Thermal sensors

Nasal pressure transducer

Inductance plethysmography

Oxygen saturation probe

Electroencephalogram (EEG)

An electroencephalogram detects electrical activity of the brain with the help of electrodes attached to the scalp. Several leads are attached to the scalp for the recording. There is a 10-20 system, internationally standardized, which helps to locate the sites on your scalp for putting electrodes.

Twenty-one electrode sites can be located using the above 10-20 system on the scalp. Reference points are decided first before putting the leads. Following are the reference points: Nasion (It is the meeting point of nasal bridge to the forehead), inion (Just beneath the occipital ridge), and two pre-auricular points.

Usually, six "exploring" electrodes and two "reference" electrodes are used to record electrical activities of the brain during polysomnography. With the help of the recording, REM and NREM stages of sleep can be readout.

Electrooculogram (EOG)

Two electrodes are used to record the cornea-positive standing potential relative to the retina.

Electrodes are placed 1 cm above and below the outer canthus of the right and left eye, respectively.

This helps to assess rapid eye movements during REM sleep.

Electromyogram (EMG)

Four electrodes are used to measure leg movements during sleep (which may be indicative of periodic limb movement disorder, PLMD).

Two leads are placed on the chin over jaw muscles, one above and one below the jawline. Two leads are placed on the leg over the anterior tibialis muscle of each leg.

These leads record muscle tone during sleep. Leg movements are recorded to diagnose periodic limb movement disorder.

Electrocardiogram (ECG)

The electrical activity of the heart is recorded with the help of electrodes to assess any abnormalities.

Thermal sensors and nasal pressure transducer record nasal and oral airflow and record interruptions in respiration.

Inductance plethysmography:

Thorax and abdominal belts record chest and abdominal movement to assess the respiratory effort during breathing.

Pulse oximetry

It detects the oxygen saturation level in blood and detects during sleep, and records fall in saturation during apnea or hypopnea.

A **sound probe** over the neck records the snoring.

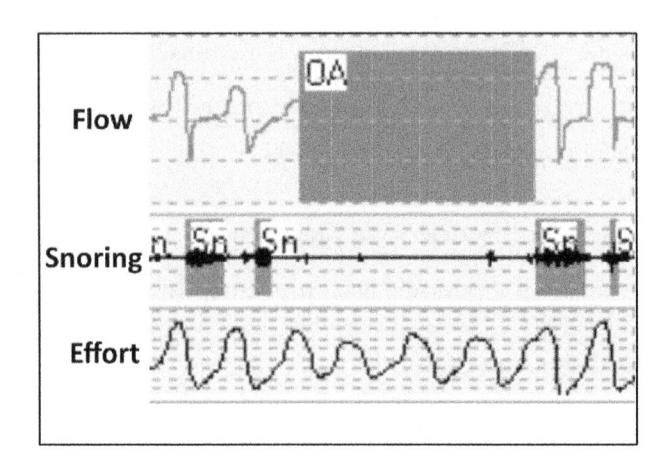

Figure 8.1: Obstructive apnea is the cessation of airflow with persistent respiratory effort

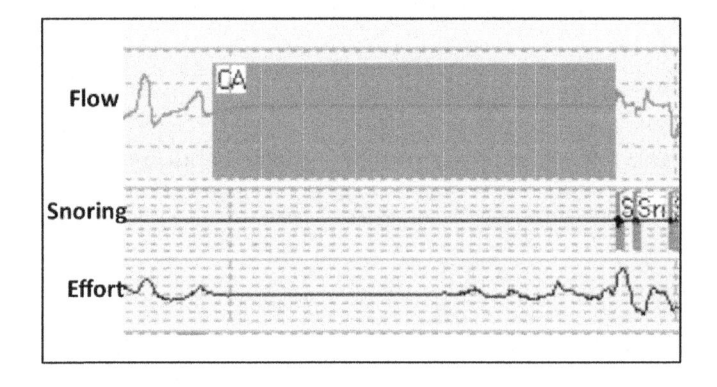

Figure 8.1: Cessation of airflow without respiratory effort

Mixed apnea is characterized by central apnea in the beginning and is followed by obstructive apnea.

Hypopnea: A ≥30% decrease in flow for ≥ 10 seconds, associated with a ≥4% oxyhemoglobin desaturation.

Respiratory event-related arousal: Arousal from sleep without meeting the criteria of hypopnea or apnea characterized by breaths with increasing effort.

In OSA patients, apnea can occur during any phase of sleep, but it is observed that apneic episodes are more prevalent during REM sleep.

Split-night PSG

It includes polysomnography followed by continuous positive airway pressure titration on the same night.

Advisable in patients with respiratory disturbance index (RDI) ≥ 40 during the initial two hours of polysomnography.

Ideally, a full night continuous positive airway pressure titration is done, but three hours of sleep is usually required for continuous positive airway pressure titration in Split-night PSG.

The AASM suggests use of portable monitors in high probability patients having no comorbidities.

Multiple Sleep Latency and Maintenance of Wakefulness Tests

It measures excessive daytime sleepiness objectively also measures maintenance of wakefulness.

This test includes multiple naps (average 4-5 naps) of 20-minutes every 2 hours during the daytime.

Latency to fall asleep is recorded and then averaged to quantify daytime sleep latency.

Normally, ≥12- 15 minutes is the daytime sleep latency time.

In Obstructive sleep apnea, sleep latencies become <10 minutes.

It cannot discriminate between OSA and narcolepsy.

The use of MSLT has decreased significantly.

Chapter 9: Consequences of OSA

OSA can be associated with the development of various systemic disorders, which broadly can be categorized into cardiovascular, neurocognitive, and metabolic sequelae.

Cardiovascular sequelae

An observational study by Marin JM et al. 2005 suggested a 2.9-fold increased rate of fatal cardiovascular events in untreated severe OSA patients.

The possible mechanism behind the development of multisystem disorders in OSA is sleep fragmentation, recurrent hypoxia causing oxidative stress, and fluctuations in intrathoracic pressure that lead to sympathetic surges and vascular endothelial dysfunction, which further eventually leads to metabolic dysregulation, hypercoagulability, and mechanical effects on the heart and vessels. A study was done by Stowhas AC, Namdar M, Biaggi P, et al., 2011 showed how obstructive apnea and hypopnea affect the aortic diameter and BP.

Hypertension

Prevalence of sleep apnea syndrome was found 30% to 40% among patients with hypertension, and similarly, about half of the patients with known OSA had coexisting hypertension.

Logan et al. studied the prevalence of unrecognized sleep apnoea in drug-resistant hypertensive patients and concluded a prevalence of 83% OSA (AHI ≥ 10 events/h). The odds ratio calculated in Sleep Heart Health Study for the presence of hypertension was 1.37.

Continuous positive airway pressure (CPAP) treatment in patients with resistant hypertension and OSA showed a reduction in mean and diastolic blood pressures and an improvement as well in the nocturnal blood pressure pattern.

A meta-analysis evaluated the effect of nocturnal nasal continuous positive airway pressure on blood pressure in obstructive sleep apnea suggested that continuous positive airway pressure (CPAP) treatment reduces blood pressure levels.

A systematic review and meta-analysis also have shown that continuous positive airway pressure (CPAP) application lowers the systolic blood pressure by 2 to 3 mm Hg in normotensive patients with obstructive sleep apnea and by 6 to 7 mm Hg in patients with resistant hypertension.

Strokes and myocardial events

A cohort study conducted by Lee CH, Sethi R, Li R, et al. showed an association between obstructive sleep apnea and cardiovascular events, particularly Stroke.

Similarly, increased rates of cardiovascular events and cardiovascular mortality were found in a large longitudinal follow-up Sleep Heart Health Study.

Prevalence of OSA was found 50% to 70% when assessed among patients with ischemic stroke. Therefore, screening for OSA in all stroke patients should be done.

Obstructive sleep apnea adversely affects the outcome of coronary artery diseases and congestive heart failure. Studies suggest OSA a significant predictor of coronary artery diseases.

Males aged 40 to 70 were 68% more likely to develop coronary artery disease if they had severe obstructive sleep apnea than no obstructive sleep apnea.

Other cardiac diseases observed in patients with obstructive sleep apnea (OSA) are cardiac arrhythmias, atrial premature contractions, ventricular ectopy.

Metabolic disturbances

OSA has been independently associated with obesity, impaired fasting glucose, hypertriglyceridemia, and reduced high-density lipoprotein (HDL). Likely mechanisms are sleep fragmentation and chronic intermittent hypoxia exposure, which trigger a systemic inflammatory response.

A study that followed patients up for ten years shows an independent association between obstructive sleep apnea and the development of metabolic diseases. So the patients with OSA should be assessed for the presence of metabolic disturbances.

Chapter 10: Management

On the basis of severity, related symptoms, and comorbidities, treatment of OSA is tailored, and it may include positive airway pressure therapy, general measures, weight loss, behavioral therapies, intraoral devices, and surgeries.

The AASM (American Academy of Sleep Medicine) considers positive airway pressure therapy as first-line therapy for sleep apnea syndrome.

General measures

Good sleep hygiene practice, avoidance of sedative-hypnotics, alcohol, and opioids.

Weight loss

Sleep AHEAD study, a randomized study conducted by Foster GD, Borradaile KE, Sanders MH, et al. assessed the association of obstructive sleep apnea among obese patients with type 2 diabetes with weight loss. After the assessment of progression and regression of sleep-disordered breathing with changes in weight, it was evidenced that changes in AHI was associated with weight loss (or weight gain) and is stronger in men than women.

A 10% reduction in weight may cause a reduction of 26% in the respiratory disturbance index as per data.

Following are the benefits of weight reduction:

- Improves RDI (respiratory disturbance index)
- Improves lung functions and blood gases
- Improves sleep hygiene
- Reduces snoring
- Improves blood pressure
- Reduces optimum CPAP pressure

Position Therapy

Position dependent sleep apnea: A condition in which AHI, while asleep, in the supine position is at least twice as in the lateral position. In such patients, lateral decubitus position may be advised for reducing the symptoms. A backpack and ball, thoracic anti-supine band, or devices that alarm the patient on changing the position can be suggested.

Weight gain causes relapse of OSA, so maintenance of weight is essential.

Noninvasive ventilation

It includes positive airway pressure with a CPAP or bilevel positive airway pressure (BiPAP).

CPAP is the standard treatment for OSA, and it generally improves this condition with and appropriate titration.

If the patient refuses nasal CPAP therapy, BiPAP or other therapies like oral appliances or different surgeries can be tried next.

All efforts should be made to improve CPAP-tolerance in patients.

Improving treatment adherence is critical to the consideration of OSA patients. Though adherence in OSA patients is similar to that in patients taking drugs, for example, statins, a group of exploration on adherence appears to have been to a great extent disregarded and should be incorporated into clinical practice.

Studies suggest improving CPAP adherence, and it must be assessed in every patient during follow-up. Adherence to oral appliances should also be assessed like CPAP.

Sleep-related breathing disorder continuum

Optimal treatment must correct OSA, upper airway resistance, and snoring. If it does not eliminate all the three problems, the symptoms that were evident at the start of the disease recur. Therefore, in the treatment of sleep-related breathing disorder, CPAP corrects OSA first, upper airway resistance next, and snoring last.

During PSG and CPAP titration, noise due to the mask leak may be interpreted as snoring and may cause inappropriate results. Therefore, differentiation between mask leak and snoring is very important. Differentiation between snoring and a CPAP mask leak can be done with the time of their production.

Mask leak occurs during expiration, while snoring occurs at peak inspiration and during the early phase of expiration.

Silent apnea- In upper airway (UA) corrective surgery, pharyngeal tissue is resected to correct snoring and apnea. But sometimes, when surgeries correct snoring but not apnea, it is known as silent apnea.

CPAP (Continuous Positive Airway Pressure) therapy

Positive Airway Pressure Therapies

CPAP works as a pneumatic splint during inspiratory and expiratory phases of respiration by delivering a fixed pressure continuously. This pressure support prevents the collapse of the upper airway during sleep.

It abolishes snoring, apneas and reduces the arousals.

Nasal CPAP therapy is the treatment of choice for OSA. It has also been found effective in mixed apneas and some central apneas.

Indication of CPAP therapy:

- Mild OSA (AHI 5-14 events/h) with associated symptoms.
- Moderate or severe OSA (AHI ≥15 events/h)
- Severe respiratory disturbance index: >20-30 irrespective of the symptoms
- Respiratory disturbance index: 5-20 with associated symptoms or comorbidities

Reduced upper airway muscle dilator activity during sleep, mainly in REM sleep, 5 to 20 cm H_2O pressure is needed to avoid collapse and associated symptoms like snoring, apnea, and oxyhemoglobin desaturation. This optimal pressure is determined during the titration polysomnogram.

Bi-level systems deliver higher pressures during inspiration and lower pressures during expiration. This can be advised in patients who report difficulty with exhaling against PAP, also.

Determining the optimal CPAP setting:

The optimal CPAP setting for home use may be defined as the minimal pressure required to resolve all apneas, hypopneas, snoring, and arousals in all stages of sleep and in all positions. Just the optimal CPAP setting should address or limit sleep apnea in supine rapid eye movement sleep to represent the impacts of gravity and changes in muscle tone that may happen in various sleep stages and positions.

Adequate titration means determining the minimum required pressure level, which abolishes hypopneas and/or apneas, oxygen desaturation, snoring, and respiratory effort-related arousals in all sleep stages and sleep positions.

A split night sleep study, in which the initial portion of the study is used to objectively document an individual's sleep-disordered breathing followed by CPAP titration during the second portion of the night, maybe indicated in certain situations.

The typical pressure in the majority of patients ranges from 5-20 cm H_2O.

There are varieties of interfaces available for the application of CPAP. Nasal masks, nasal inserts, or full-face masks are some of the variants. A well-fitting interface is required to ensure that there are no air leaks.

CPAP device has the following parts: (Figure 10.1)

A motor and humidifier: Motor generates a continuous positive-pressure by blowing air in the tubing attached. A humidifier increases the moisture in the air produced by the motor to avoid dryness and discomfort.

Tube: It is a flexible plastic tube that carries the air generated by the device and delivers it to the patient through a mask attached to its other end.

Mask: There are several masks available. The main purpose is to seal the nose, mouth, or both properly to avoid any leak.

The pressure generated by CPAP keeps the airway patent by increasing the retroglossal, retropalatal and lateral spaces (by thinning out the lateral pharyngeal wall) of the upper airway.

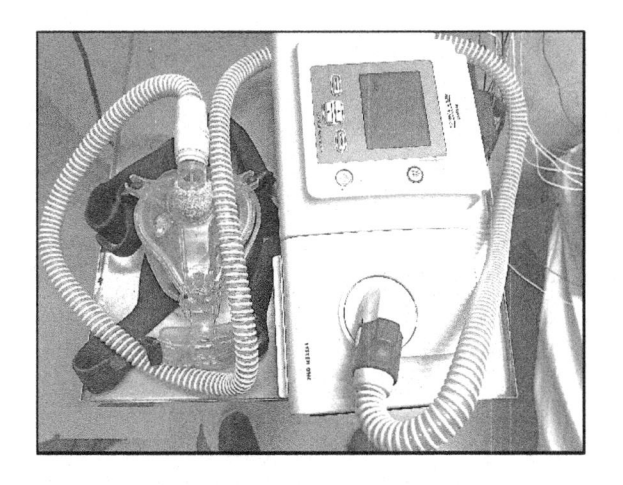

Figure 10.1: CPAP device

There are two types of CPAP devices:

1. Auto-CPAP: Pressure varies automatically as per need over the course of sleep. The pressure required to keep the airway patent during different stages and in different positions of sleep varies. This device detects the change and adjusts the pressure automatically.

2. Manual/fixed CPAP: Pressure is set manually before the application of the device, and it remains fixed during the course of sleep.

There has been observed marginal better compliance of patients towards auto CPAP than fixed CPAP.

Effectiveness

Studies have observed that CPAP application in OSA patients:

    Improves systemic hypertension

Improves left ventricular ejection fraction

Improves right-side heart function

Improves pulmonary hypertension

Lowers risk for Stroke

Lowers risk for diabetes

Improves quality of life

Improves neurocognitive symptoms like attentiveness and concentration

Adherence

Follow-up evaluation is a must to ensure CPAP adherence and response monitoring.

Unfortunately, many patients do not adhere to CPAP therapy.

Objective measurement of compliance and adherence can be done by machine-on and mask-on times recorded. These data can be downloaded and assessed by the physician.

Use of device for more than 4 hours/night for 5-7 nights/week is generally considered compliant.

In poorly adherent patients, mask interface, leakage, humidification, and sleep hygiene should be assessed.

Complications and adverse effects

Abdominal discomfort due to aerophagia

Chest discomfort,

Claustrophobia- nasal pillows can be used.

Conjunctivitis

Difficulty in breathing (mostly during the expiratory phase): A ramp setting can be used to avoid this problem. This setting starts the device at lower pressure and then gradually increases the optimal pressure over a predetermined period.

Difficulty in falling asleep

Dryness: Humidification improves this condition.

Epistaxis

Nasal congestion- Antihistamines and corticosteroids are advised.

Nasal dryness- Saline sprays can be used.

Rash

Rhinorrhea

Skin abrasions

BPAP therapy (Bi-level Positive Airway Pressure)

Bi-level Positive Airway Pressure delivers a constant pressure during both the inspiratory and expiratory phase of respiration.

EPAP (expiratory positive airway pressure) abolishes apneas, and the IPAP (inspiratory positive airway pressure) abolishes hypopneas during sleep.

BPAP device also has similar parts as CPAP. It also contains a motor and humidifier, tube, and mask-like CPAP device.

Patients who show intolerance to high CPAP pressures are advised BiPAP.

Generally, BiPAP is advised when a patient needs a pressure >15 cm water.

Oral appliances

There are various oral appliances. They increase upper airway caliber by pulling the tongue forward, moving mandible and soft palate anteriorly, and expanding the posterior airspace to reduce obstruction during sleep. The anticipated outcome of oral appliances treatment includes improvement of the signs and symptoms, decrease in AHI, and improvement in oxygen saturation.

Genioglossus is the primary muscle along with other muscles of the pharyngeal airway wall, which influences the airway caliber the most when the jaw is opened.

Oral appliances thin the lateral pharyngeal walls and increase the caliber.

Examples of oral appliances:

- Mandibular advancement/ repositioner devices- Mandibular repositioner devices are adjustable and are usually preferred. Adjustable mandibular repositioners are relatively more efficacious than nonadjustable mandibular repositioner.
- Palatal lifting devices
- Tongue retaining device (TRD)

Indications:

- Patients with mild-to-moderate OSA, not giving consent for CPAP devices.
- Patients with mild-to-moderate OSA, not responding to CPAP therapy.
- Patients with mild-to-moderate OSA with CPAP therapy failure
- Severe OSA- Initial trial of CPAP is given as oral appliances therapy is less effective.

Contraindications:

- <6-10 teeth in each arch
- Inability to open jaw widely

- Inability to protrude mandible forward
- Temporomandibular joint dysfunction
- Using dentures
- Bruxism

The application of oral appliances needs a thorough multidisciplinary evaluation by a sleep specialist and a dental specialist.

Following are the key variables that increase the efficacy of oral appliances:

1. Mild-to-moderate OSA

2. Mandibular repositioner protrusion distance >70% of baseline

3. AHI in supine position > AHI in lateral sleep position

4. Low BMI

5. Younger age

6. Small neck circumference

7. Short soft palate

8. Regular follow up and adjustment, as needed

Studies have reported CPAP therapy as superior to oral appliances therapy.

Adherence rates are not as well defined in oral appliances as in CPAP because CPAP devices can record the data, which can be used as feedback, while in oral appliances, voluntary reporting is needed, which is subjective and quite unreliable. This is too one of the reasons for its limited use in clinical practice.

Complications:

- Temporomandibular joint disorders
- Too much salivation
- Dental injuries
- Bite change
- Gum irritation
- Occlusal changes
- Myofascial pain

Surgical Approaches

There are varieties of surgeries available for reducing the collapsibility or increasing the airway caliber.

Nasal surgeries

    Septoplasty

    Sinus surgery

Oral surgeries

    Tonsillectomy ± adenoidectomy

- Lingular tonsillectomy
- Uvulopalatopharyngoplasty (UPPP)
- Tissue reduction surgery
- Genioglossus advancement with hyoid myotomy (GAHM)
- Sliding genioplasty
- Maxillomandibular osteotomy [MMO].

Tracheostomy

Surgical procedures chosen for a patient is based upon the level of obstruction. Phase 1 surgeries aim at reducing obstruction at the nasal, lingual, or palatal levels. Maxillomandibular advancement (MMA) is a Phase 2 surgery.

Septoplasty and turbinate reduction, leading to an improvement in nasal patency and a lesser nasal continuous positive airway pressure (CPAP) requirement, are the most commonly performed surgeries.

Tonsillectomy and adenoidectomy are useful as primary therapy in children with OSA; however, it is not as helpful as in adults.

Uvulopalatopharyngoplasty (UPPP) with or without tonsillectomy is also done, but a systematic review noted that this surgery as a sole surgical procedure does not have a consistent effect on the AHI. Therefore this cannot be recommended as a stand-alone treatment for obstructive sleep apnea.

UPPP and MMA are multilevel surgical approaches and need good skill.

Laser-assisted uvulopalatoplasty (LAUP) is done by a carbon dioxide laser, which removes the uvula and a part of the soft palate.

There are minimally invasive techniques also like radiofrequency volumetric tissue reduction. It is an advanced technique that is used to treat turbinate hypertrophy and to reduce the size of the base of the tongue, which eventually reduces the collapse and improves the symptoms of obstructive sleep apnea.

Palatal implants are used to stiffen the soft palate, which protects the upper airway from collapse.

Genioglossus advancement with hyoid myotomy moves the tongue forward without disturbing the mandible. Performing this surgery helps in achieving a larger-caliber airway.

The success percentage of such combination surgeries are variable and may range from 23% to 77%.

There are inconsistent results and increased surgical risks in genioglossus advancement and related surgeries. Due to which these surgeries are not recommended nowadays as a therapy for sleep-disordered breathing.

Surgical Correction of the Upper Airway

On the basis of site of obstruction, patients of sleep-disordered breathing can be classified into the following categories:

Type I- Retropalatal obstruction- UPPP is usually the preferred corrective surgery.

Type II- Retropalatal and Retroglossal obstruction- MMO is usually the preferred corrective surgery as it can correct obstruction at all levels.

Type III- Retroglossal obstruction- GAHM is usually the preferred corrective surgery.

Indications:

- Patients with mild-to-moderate OSA, not giving consent for CPAP devices, oral appliances, or other medical therapy.
- Patients with mild-to-moderate OSA, not responding to CPAP therapy oral appliances or other noninvasive medical therapy.
- Patients with mild-to-moderate OSA with CPAP or other treatment failures
- Abnormal growth or mass lesions in the upper airway

There may be a need for multiple surgeries for correction. Even there may be a need for CPAP therapy as well, post-surgery.

Surgeries in multiple phases are suggested by Riley-Powell-Stanford surgical protocol. According to this protocol, UPPP and GAHM procedures are done in phase I, followed by phase II, which includes MMO procedure if the patient is not relieved.

As mentioned above, UPPP is usually the preferred corrective surgery for Type I obstruction, GAHM for type III obstruction. In type II obstruction, UPPP and GAHM are both performed as per Riley-Powell-Stanford surgical protocol.

Uvulopalatopharyngoplasty (UPPP):

It includes surgical resection of the uvula, soft palate, and pharyngeal tissue. It may or may not include tonsillectomy.

Weight gain may cause recurrence after this surgery.

Uvulopalatopharyngoglossoplasty (UPPPG) is a modified version of the surgery, which includes surgical resection of the base of the tongue also.

Complications:

- Change in voice
- Difficulty/ Pain on deglutition
- Hemorrhage
- Loss of taste or sensory nerves of the tongue
- Nasopharyngeal stenosis
- Silent apnea
- Speech difficulties

Maxillomandibular osteotomy

Mandible and palate are repositioned forward in order to increases tension of genioglossus muscle and to increases retroglossal space. This surgery is done in phase II for correction of obstruction as per Riley-Powell-Stanford surgical protocol.

Bariatric surgery

- Bariatric surgery has shown a decrease in AHI in OSAS.
- An adjunct to positive airway pressure therapy

The exact localization of the site of obstruction is important and can be assessed by MRI (magnetic resonance imaging), CT (computed tomography) imaging, endoscopy, and lateral cephalometry.

Medications

To date, so many pharmacologic agents have been trialed for the primary treatment of obstructive sleep apnea. But none have shown a significant benefit in the treatment of obstructive sleep apnea.

Modafinil, also known as and armodafinil, improves fatigue and daytime wakefulness in excessive residual sleepiness without disturbing normal sleep architecture.

It is seen that in patients who still remain symptomatic despite giving optimized treatment for sleep-disordered breathing, Modafinil, a stimulant, can be utilized as adjunctive therapy. The dose of Modafinil ranges from 200 to 400 mg daily.

Solriamfetol, a Dopamine/norepinephrine reuptake inhibitor (DNRI) and was approved in 2019, and it also helps in improving daytime sleepiness in patients with excessive residual sleepiness.

PAP therapy, despite the use of humidification, sometimes can cause or exacerbate rhinitis. In that situation, topical nasal corticosteroids have shown effectiveness as an adjunctive therapy to treat rhinitis.

Residual excessive sleepiness

A small percentage of the patient might present with such a condition.

Residual excessive sleepiness is defined in an adequately treated patient and is characterized by an ESS score of ≥11 during follow-up CPAP visits.

Adequate treatment is characterized by:

    A residual AHI < 15/hr

    Using CPAP more than 3 hrs/day

    Depression score < 7 without any antidepressant

Complex sleep apnea syndrome:

This syndrome is characterized by central apneas, which persist and comprise more than half of the residual sleep-disordered breathing when obstructive events have disappeared with PAP therapy. And it must be more than five events/hour. The exact criteria for diagnosis and exact pathophysiology behind the development of complex sleep apnea syndrome are still to be established.

All causes of excessive sleepiness even after CPAP therapy must be assessed before labeling residual sleepiness syndrome.

>   Adequacy of titration

>   Any other sleep disorder like narcolepsy or periodic limb movement disorder

>   CPAP Compliance (good compliance means the use of CPAP for > 4 hours and ≥5 nights/week)

>   Neurologic conditions

>   Shift worker

>   Use of medications causing sleepiness- narcotics, antihistamines, tricyclic antidepressants, benzodiazepines.

Chapter: 11 Prevention

Prevention

Weight reduction

Regular exercise

Maintenance of sleep hygiene

Position alarm- monitors the position and ring on change of position.

Tennis ball/ pillow- kept at the back of the patient, which maintains the patient head and neck in position and keeps the upper airway patent.

Avoid caffeine before sleep.

Avoidance of alcohol and sedatives- alcohol and sedatives cause depression and worsen apnea.

Avoidance of smoking- Studies have reported an increase in daytime somnolence in smokers.

Chapter 12: Follow up

A regular follow-up is important during treatment.

Patients start improving after the application of CPAP. Assessment of the efficacy of the treatment, compliance, and treatment-related complications is important, and for this reason, regular follow-up is important.

Follow up at every 2 to 3-month intervals is usually advised.

Repeat CPAP titrations are only performed when the patient is not showing relief or there is a recurrence of symptoms.

Counseling to the patient and the family members plays an important role. It improves compliance and gives psychological support to the patient and family.

Chapter 13: Role of yoga

Introduction:

This was originated long back in India.

It is a practice that includes breathing techniques, physical activities, and mental exercises.

Yoga is not an alternative for medical treatment.

Yoga can be beneficial in addition to medical therapy for sleep apnea.

Yoga strengthens and increases the tone of pharyngeal muscles and decreases the chances of upper airway collapse during sleep.

Yoga improves the lifestyle, sleep hygiene, and diminishes stress.

Following exercises are helpful in sleep apnea.

1. Cat-Cow

Cow position (Figure 13.1)

Bend down on your hands and knees with a flat back.

Shoulders should be above your hands.

Hips should be above your knees.

Start a deep and slow inhalation.

Curve your back towards the floor and lift the chin up in order to keep your neck and spine in a line.

Relax your abdomen while hanging down to the floor.

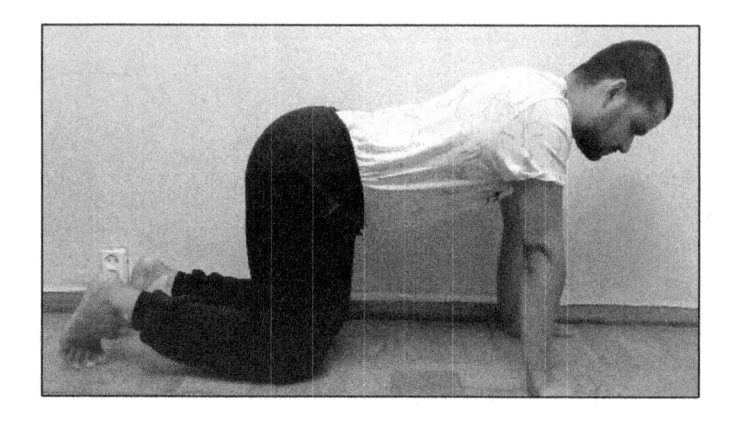

Figure 13.1: Cow position

Cat position (Figure 13.2)

Start slow exhalation.

Curve your spine back towards the ceiling and bring your head/chin down towards the floor.

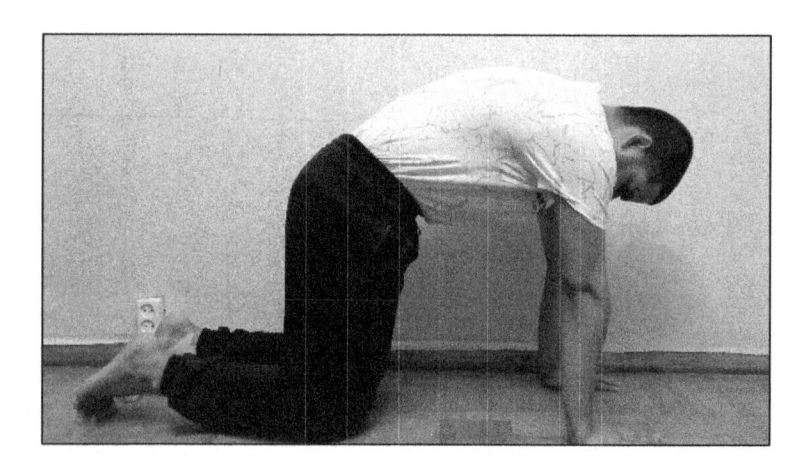

Figure 13.1: Cat position

Caution:

Aggressive/forceful practice of this exercise might lead to cervical or spinal injuries.

Avoid doing this exercise in few conditions like backache or spondylitis, neck stiffness, etc.

2. Anuloma Viloma (Nadhi Sodhana)

Breathing via each nostril alternatively is practiced. (Figure 13.3)

It calms the mind and diminishes stress.

It is useful in improving concentration.

Sit with your back straight.

Slowly exhale air out of your lungs as much as possible.

Close one of the nostrils, suppose right with the thumb of the right hand and inhale deep and slow as much as possible through the other one, i.e., left nostril.

Now close the left nostril also using the ring finger of the right hand, keeping your right nostril closed with the thumb, and hold the breath for few seconds.

Open the right nostril by releasing the thumb and exhale slowly as much as possible through your right nostril while keeping the left nostril closed by the ring finger of the right hand.

Inhale through the open right nostril deep and slowly while keeping the left nostril closed by the ring finger of the right hand.

Close the right nostril by using the thumb of the right hand and hold the breath for few seconds.

Now open the left nostril by releasing the ring finger and exhale slowly and as much as possible through your left nostril while keeping the right nostril closed by the thumb of the right hand.

This completes a cycle of Anuloma Viloma.

Try to perform at least ten cycles daily.

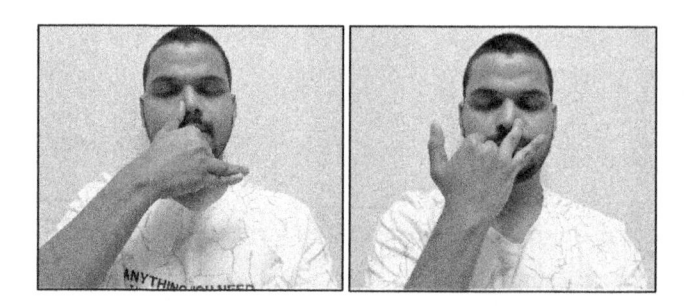

Figure 13.3: Anulom Vilom

3. Ujjayi (Hissing Breath / Ocean's Breath/ Victorious Breath/ Warrior Breath/) (Figure 13.4)

Inhale deeply and slowly first.

Forceful exhalation through nostrils against a pressure produces a hissing sound. This pressure is created by constricting the throat during exhalation. Try to involve your abdominal muscles also during exhalation.

It is suggested that ujjayi increases the tone of the pharyngeal muscles and thus decreases the chances of the collapse of the upper airway during sleep.

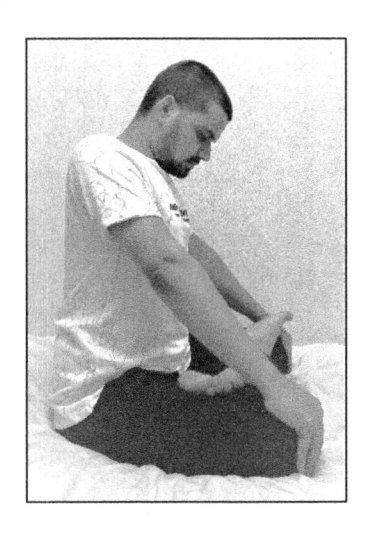

Figure 13.4: Ujjayi

Caution:

Avoid doing if there is an incisional hernia or just after major surgeries.

4. Mrigi Mudra

Mriga means "Deer."

Mudra means "Position."

Sit with a straight back.

Rest left palm on your left knee.

Fold right index finger and middle finger.

Keep thumb, ring finger, and little fingers open and straight.

Close the right nostril with the right thumb and inhale deeply through the left nostril.

Wait for few seconds or can count up to 5 or 10 during inhalation.

Now close the left nostril using the ring and small finger of the right hand.

Wait for few seconds or can count up to 5 or 10 during inhalation.

Release the thumb and exhale through the right nostril.

Wait for few seconds or can count up to 5 or 10 during inhalation.

This completes one cycle.

Repeat the cycle with the left hand.

5. Bhastrika Pranayama (Bellow's Breath) (Figure 13.5)

Bhastrika is a process of rapid and forceful inhalation and exhalation using abdominal muscles.

Sit straight with your back straight.

Take few small breaths.

Inhale deeply and exhale forcefully.

Wait for 1 or 2 seconds, then again inhale deeply.

This completes one cycle.

Repeat the cycle several times.

You can divide the exercise into 3 phases. In the first phase, do ten cycles and relax. In the second phase, do 20 cycles and relax. In the third phase, do 30 cycles and relax.

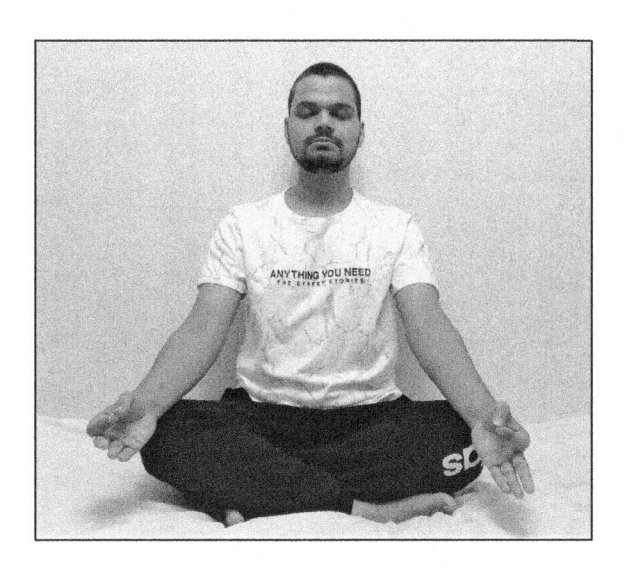

Figure 13.5: Bhastrika

Caution:

Avoid doing this exercise during pregnancy.

Stop doing the exercise if you feel lightheaded.

6. Seated Forward Bend

Sit with your back straight and legs extended.

Inhale deeply.

Extend your arms over your head.

Wait for few seconds.

Bend forward and exhale.

Hold the position for 10 seconds.

Sit back straight and inhale.

This completes one cycle.

Repeat the cycle several times.

Chapter 14: Role of reflexology acupressure and acupuncture

Acupuncture:

The traditional practice of Chinese medicine

Fine thin needles are inserted into the specific areas of the body through the skin.

Needles inserted through the skin cause micro-injuries and vasodilation, which increases blood supply to that region. This facilitates healing. It also stimulates the nerves, which in response release neuropeptides to cause analgesia.

Acupressure:

It is also a traditional practice of Chinese medicine.

Acupressure is also based on a similar principle as acupuncture.

Reflexology:

This is a technique that basically involves the application of pressure onto the ears, feet, and **hands**.

The concept behind this is that different areas of the foot have connections with the rest of the body. The application of pressure on those areas brings an effect on that particular organ system.

These treatment methods are an alternative therapy for sleep apnea.

Acupressure points for sleep apnea:
GV16 (Governing Vessel 16) (Figure 14.1)
It is located just below the base of the skull in the midline.

Stimulation of this point using the middle finger relieves insomnia and improves the quality of sleep.

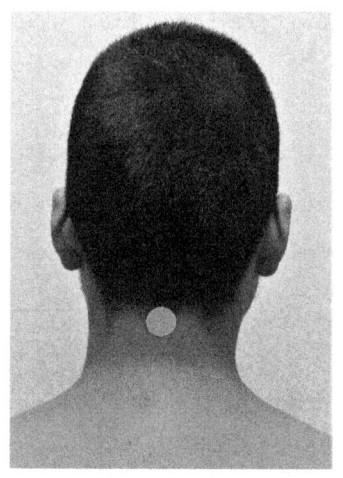

Figure 14.1: GV 16 Acupressure point

Point B38 (Figure 14.2)
It is located between the medial scapular border and the spine on both sides.

Stimulation of B38 is also helpful in the treatment of other respiratory problems like cough and dyspnea.

The patient is asked to lie down supine on the ground, and two tennis balls are kept bilaterally beneath point B38.

The patient breathes slowly and deeply for 2 minutes.

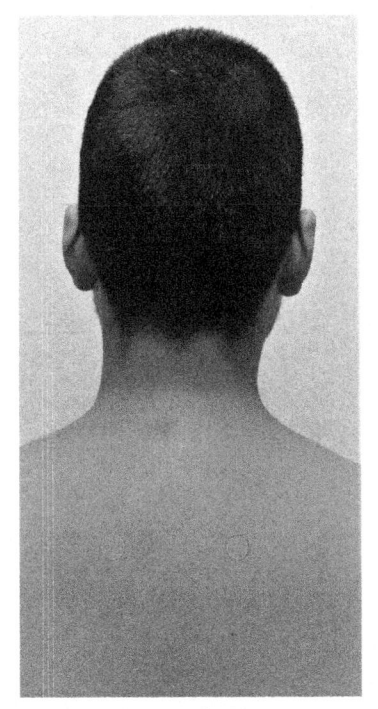

Figure 14.2: B 38 Acupressure point

H7 (Heart 7) (Figure 14.3)
Also known as the Spirit Gate.

It is located at the medial border of the distal forearm over the wrist crease.

Relieves insomnia

This point can be pressed by the thumb.

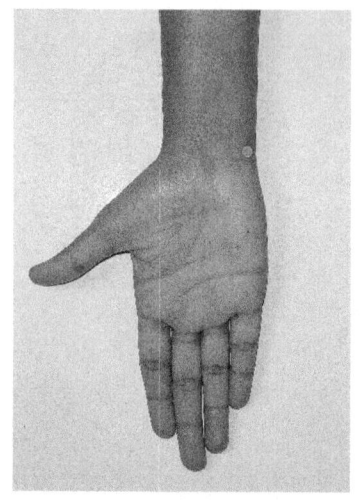

Figure 14.3: H7 Acupressure point

Point P6 (Pericardium 6) (Figure 14.4)
Also known as Inner Gate point.

This point is located anteriorly on the midline of the forearm, three fingers above the proximal crease of the wrist.

It helps in treating anxiety, indigestion, nausea, and vomiting, which in response improve the quality of sleep.

This point also has a beneficial effect on respiratory conditions like cough and dyspnea.

Stimulation of this point can be done by using the thumb.

This point is pressed firmly by the thumb for a minute and then released.

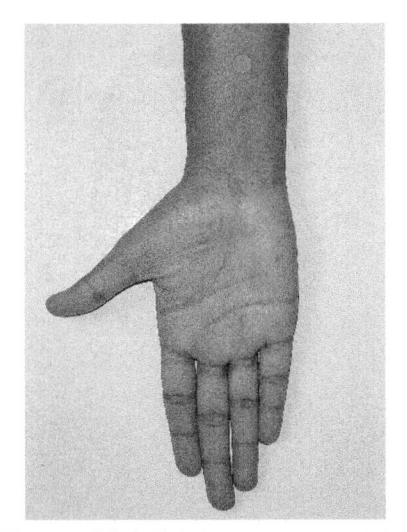

Figure 14.4: P6 Acupressure point

B10 (Bladder10) (Figure 14.5)
This point is located approx. 1.5 inches below the base of the skull on the sides of the spine bilaterally.

Stimulation of this point improves the quality of sleep.

It improves upper airway infections like nasal congestion and sore throat.

These points can be stimulated by the pulp of fingers.

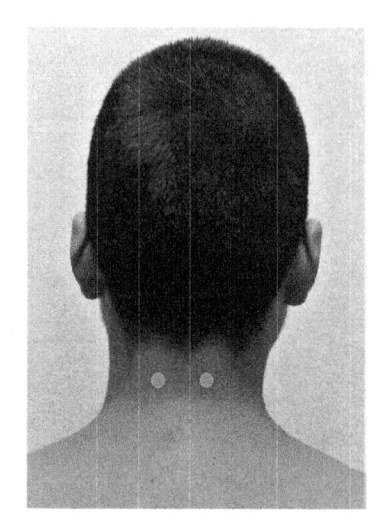

Figure 14.5: B10 Acupressure point